AF379431

THE BURNOUT PARAMEDIC

REMEDY & PREVENTION

Darrell V. Maxwell

THE BURNOUT PARAMEDIC

REMEDY & PREVENTION

A systematic way for paramedics to communicate with each other in dealing with the issues they face as paramedics.

ISBN 978-0-7414-2792-2

Published by:

INFINITY
PUBLISHING.COM
1094 New Dehaven Street, Suite 100
West Conshohocken, PA 19428-2713
Info@buybooksontheweb.com
www.buybooksontheweb.com
Toll-free (877) BUY BOOK
Local Phone (610) 941-9999
Fax (610) 941-9959

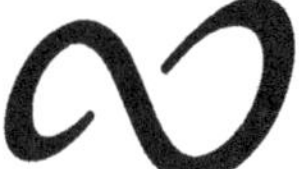

Printed in the United States of America

Published August 2013

Table of Contents

Purpose of This Course

The Burnout Paramedic: Remedy & Prevention

The purpose of this course:

To provide help for paramedics who are burned out.

To provide help for paramedics who are on the road to becoming burned out.

To provide help for paramedics who do not want to become burned out.

How will this course help paramedics?

By providing a systematic way for paramedics to communicate with their coworkers in dealing with the issues they face as paramedics.

An Interview with the Author

An Interview with the Author

Share with your readers a little about yourself.

My name is Darrell V. Maxwell, and I have been a fire & rescue officer with the city of Dallas, Texas, for the past 15½ years. I became a paramedic in May of 1991.

Why did you decide to become a fire & rescue officer?

My decision to become a fire & rescue officer began as a result of my volunteer work with the American Red Cross. I enjoyed teaching First Aid & CPR classes. My desire to become a paramedic started when I wanted to advance my First Aid & CPR skills. To be a 911 paramedic in the city of Dallas, you have to be a firefighter also. That is how I became a fire & rescue officer.

Your book is titled **The Burnout Paramedic: Remedy & Prevention.** ***What inspired you to write this book?***

For one thing, I never would have imagined that I would be a victim of burnout. After all, the reason why I joined the fire department was to become a paramedic. I remember watching the TV show *911* and role-playing by being a paramedic using the scenarios I saw on TV. During my ambulance rotations and as a rookie paramedic, I would evaluate the runs I made and practice how I would perform if I were to experience those same runs in the field again. I really wanted to be a good paramedic.

Did you become a good paramedic?

After about two years, I felt comfortable on the ambulance. After three years, I reached a point where I was able to be calm and confident in performing my job in crisis situations.

How did you become a burned out paramedic?

Prior to my research on the subject, "burnout," I didn't know how I became burned out. You are looking at someone who was excited about being a paramedic. I looked forward to the critical and challenging situations I faced on the ambulance. I also enjoyed sharing my knowledge and experiences with paramedic interns and rookie paramedics. Anytime we had a critical patient, I was the one who wanted to ride in the back, even if it was my turn to drive. I also was happy about the fact that I lived 5 minutes from my station, and my daughter went to school right down the street. At this point in my career, I had every reason to believe I would be a paramedic my entire career with the Dallas Fire & Rescue department.

An Interview with the Author

What was the result of your research?

I experienced a traumatic run that changed my life. When I returned to the station after the run, I laid down and I was afraid to close my eyes. They called the chaplain to come and talk to me. The next shift, I participated in a debriefing at the hospital in which everyone that treated the patients took part. After the debriefing, this was all the help I received. So I dealt with my emotions the best way I knew how.

Did you ever recover from this traumatic run?

Over time, I noticed a change in my attitude towards being a paramedic. I found it hard to deal with runs that were not emergencies. I began to lose my excitement for the job. I found myself complaining a lot about the job. I got to the point where I did not want to be a paramedic anymore.

Why didn't you talk to someone about how you felt?

The paramedics whom I worked with were unable to share with me what I needed to hear that would encourage me to remain a paramedic. I reached the point of no return. I wanted off the ambulance.

What did you do once you were removed from the EMS system?

Two years later, my paramedic certification was about to expire and I was deciding if I should renew it. I began to look back to find out what happened. How did I get to be a burnout? I really wanted to be a paramedic. It was at this time I began to research burnout and stress on the job. I found out that there were not many books that dealt specifically with the problems that paramedics face on the job. I did find some articles on the Internet, but not much.

Is this when you began to write your book?

The books that I read on the topic of burnout were geared for the professions of lawyers, schoolteachers, social workers, therapists, nurses, doctors, and police. After reading and meditating on the material through the eyes of a paramedic, this is how I came up with the book *The Burnout Paramedic: Remedy & Prevention.*

An Interview with the Author

Who will benefit from your book?

The paramedics who will find this book helpful are those who:

> No longer desire to be a paramedic
>
> No longer enjoy being a paramedic
>
> No longer are excited about being a paramedic
>
> No longer feel the job of a paramedic is a challenge
>
> Have trouble getting along with their partner on the ambulance
>
> Are unable to cope with the problems experienced on the ambulance
>
> Have not recovered from a traumatic run made on the ambulance
>
> Want to quit their job as a paramedic, but can't afford to
>
> Want to quit their job as a paramedic, but don't have another job to fall back on
>
> Want to transfer to another position, but it is not happening
>
> Don't know where to go to get help for the problems they are experiencing on the ambulance and
>
> Have a negative attitude towards the ambulance.

This book will also be beneficial to those paramedics who:

> Don't believe that they will ever become a burnout paramedic
>
> Don't believe that they will ever become tired of the ambulance and
>
> Don't believe that they will ever stop caring about people.

The Remedy to Burnout

The Remedy to Burnout

1. **First recognize that you are suffering from burnout.**

   A. Must acknowledge that you have a problem.

   B. Responding to the First Session of Questions and Are You a Burnout? will help you realize if you are burned out.

2. **Secondly, you must make the decision that you still want to be a paramedic.**

   A. Once you have made this decision, then you will look for ways to deal with the problems you are having as a paramedic.

   B. Responding to Is It Time For a Job Change? will help you make your decision.

   C. If after responding to the Is It Time for a Job Change? questions, you decide that you will quit your job as a paramedic:

   Discuss the matter with the paramedic counselor at this time.

3. **Third, once the decision has been made that you want to be a paramedic and that you desire help:**

   Respond to the questions in The Agreement, Second Session of Questions, Preparation for Discussion, and Solution Finder.

4. **Fourth, the key to recovery from burnout will take place as paramedics help paramedics:**

   This is done by taking part in the discussion sessions' outlines in the First Monthly Meeting, Second Monthly Meeting, Third Monthly Meeting, Fourth Monthly Meeting, Fifth Monthly Meeting, and Sixth Monthly Meeting.

5. **Fifth, in order to stay on track and keep the discussion sessions from becoming a gripe session:**

   A. All suggestions, questions, comments, etc., must be given with the attitude of helping.

   B. The paramedic counselor is responsible for making sure all suggestions, questions, comments, etc., are given with the attitude of helping by:

   1. Asking the paramedic giving the suggestions, questions, comments, etc., the reason(s) for his/her response.

   2. Observing that if the suggestions, questions, comments, etc., will not be helpful, it will not be allowed.

How to Use This Workbook

How to Use This Workbook

1.   The purpose of the questions contained in this workbook are:

    A.   To help you to search out how you truly feel in order to pinpoint the cause of why you are burned out, if you are. Once we know the reason why, then we can focus on the solution.

    B.   To help you to see your shortcomings as a paramedic.

    C.   To help you to admit when you are wrong.

    D.   To help you to think clearly about your problems as a paramedic, so that you will be able to receive help for your situation.

    E.   To encourage you to think about why you really want to be a paramedic.

2.   Below are the suggested approaches to be taken with the questions in this workbook:

    A.   Answer each question in detail.

    B.   Spend time thinking about your response to all of the questions, before you answer.

    C.   If you come to a question that you do not have an immediate response to, skip it and come back to it later.

    D.   If you find yourself giving similar answers to some of the questions, it's okay. Continue on.

    E.   It is very important that you answer each question as detailed as possible because:

        1.   It will help you in making decisions in relation to your career as a paramedic.

        2.   It will help other paramedics during the discussion phase of this course.

3.   Points to remember while using this workbook:

    A.   For this workbook to help you, you must be honest in answering these questions.

    B.   No one will see your answers but you. So be sincere in your response to the questions.

    C.   Do not be concerned if you find yourself writing similar answers to the questions.

        This means that you will be able to clearly see your situation.

    D.   Some questions are worded in a manner to bring you to answer a specific question. Example: Do you want to be a paramedic? Yes or No

    E.   There are no correct or incorrect answers to these questions. The key is to express how you truly feel.

First Session of Questions

First Session of Questions

1. List the reasons why you look forward to going to work to perform your duties as a paramedic.

____
____
____
____
____

2. List the reasons why you enjoy helping people as a paramedic.

____
____
____
____
____

3. List the reasons why other paramedics like being your partner on the ambulance.

____
____
____
____
____

4. List the reasons why you do not dislike riding the ambulance.

____
____
____
____
____

5. List three recent incidents when you showed compassion to your patients.

____
____
____
____
____

First Session of Questions

6.   List the reasons why you want to remain a paramedic.

7.   Explain why you do not get depressed when you think about your job as a paramedic.

8.   Why does being a paramedic mean more to you than just another job that pays the bills?

9.   List as many aspects of your job as a paramedic that you like.

10.   List the reasons why you chose to become a paramedic.

First Session of Questions

11. Why don't you get upset when citizens call for an ambulance for matters that are not an emergency?

12. How do you keep from getting impatient with patients who call on a regular basis?

13. How do you keep from getting angry with patients who wait until after 12:00 a.m. to call for matters that could have been taken care of during the daytime?

14. How do you respond when the doctors and nurses show how glad they are when you bring patients to their hospitals?

15. How are you able to work aggressive CPR on a person who is obviously (based on medical history or trauma) not going to be restored to life?

First Session of Questions

16.   What keeps you from complaining about your job as a paramedic?

17.   List the reasons why the average person can perform the duties of a paramedic.

18.   List the reasons why you do not need help with the problems you are having as a paramedic.

19.   List the aspects of the process of keeping your paramedic certification that you feel are beneficial to you performing your job as a paramedic.

20.   Are there paramedics who you are not happy about riding the ambulance with? List the reasons why you feel this way.

21. Why haven't you discussed with the paramedic(s) the reasons why you do not want to ride the ambulance with them?

22. List the reasons why you are able to consistently show compassion towards your patients.

23. List the reasons why you do not believe that you are burned out as a paramedic.

24. Do you conduct yourself in a manner that will cause a paramedic who is experiencing burnout to feel comfortable coming to you for help? Give the reason for your answer.

25. How are you able to keep a positive attitude when you ride the ambulance, despite the fact you did not get a good night's rest prior to coming to work?

Are You a Burnout?

Are You a Burnout?

	Yes	No
Have you lost interest in your job as a paramedic?	_______	_______
Are you frustrated with your job as a paramedic?	_______	_______
Is it correct to conclude that you are no longer motivated to do a good job as a paramedic?	_______	_______
In relation to your duties as a paramedic, would you consider yourself as a negative thinker?	_______	_______
Is it correct to conclude that it is no longer a challenge to perform your duties as a paramedic?	_______	_______
Is your job as a paramedic boring to you?	_______	_______
Do you feel your job, as a paramedic, is going nowhere?	_______	_______
Do you dread going to work to perform your duties as a paramedic?	_______	_______
Are you just going through the motions performing your duties as a paramedic?	_______	_______
Do you feel like you are overwhelmed by the problems of others in performing your duties as a paramedic?	_______	_______
Have you lost your enthusiasm to be a paramedic?	_______	_______
Have you lost your purpose as a paramedic?	_______	_______
Would you say you are no longer dedicated to your job as a paramedic?	_______	_______
Would you say you no longer care about your job as a paramedic?	_______	_______

Are You a Burnout?

	Yes	No
Do you find yourself griping about your job as a paramedic?	_________	_________
Do you see yourself as a failure as a paramedic?	_________	_________
Do you become angry because you have to perform your duties as a paramedic?	_________	_________
Have you lost the ambition you had when you first became a paramedic?	_________	_________
Are you disillusioned as a paramedic?	_________	_________
Is it correct to conclude that your job as a paramedic is no longer satisfying your expectations?	_________	_________
Do you see yourself as helpless as a paramedic?	_________	_________
Would you say that you are depressed as a paramedic?	_________	_________
Do you see yourself as irresponsible as a paramedic?	_________	_________
Do you see yourself as exhausted as a paramedic?	_________	_________
Do you see yourself as lackadaisical as a paramedic?	_________	_________
Do you show little concern for your job as a paramedic?	_________	_________
Do you find yourself angry with paramedics who want to do a good job?	_________	_________
Do you find yourself full of cynicism as a paramedic?	_________	_________
Do you find yourself lacking motivation as a paramedic?	_________	_________

Are You a Burnout?

	Yes	No
Have you lately lost your appetite to eat?	_________	_________
Have you lately not been getting much sleep?	_________	_________
Have you been isolating yourself from friends?	_________	_________
Do you see yourself withdrawing from relatives and immediate family?	_________	_________
Have you been quarrelsome lately?	_________	_________
Have you lost your desire to achieve as a paramedic?	_________	_________
Do you find it hard to tolerate people at work?	_________	_________
Is it correct to conclude that you have lost compassion for people because of your job as a paramedic?	_________	_________
Are you miserable as a paramedic?	_________	_________
Are you ready to change jobs?	_________	_________
Are you callous as a paramedic?	_________	_________
Are you disappointed with the way things have turned out as a paramedic?	_________	_________
Do you find yourself being cruel to patients?	_________	_________
Do you find yourself being rude to the family and friends of your patients?	_________	_________
Are you tired of your job as a paramedic?	_________	_________
Do you hate your job as a paramedic?	_________	_________
Have you lost your sensitivity as a paramedic?	_________	_________

Are You a Burnout?

	Yes	No
Is it correct to conclude that you have lost empathy because of your job as a paramedic?	__________	__________
Are you no longer able to place yourself in the shoes of others in order to understand and share in people's experiences?	__________	__________
Do you see yourself disliking people / patients?	__________	__________
Is it correct to conclude that you are no longer committed to your job as a paramedic?	__________	__________
Do you dislike your job as a paramedic?	__________	__________
Is it correct to conclude that you are giving the minimum, rather than giving your all, in your duties as a paramedic?	__________	__________
Do you lack the emotional energy to handle everyday hassles calmly?	__________	__________
Are you overwhelmed with your job as a paramedic?	__________	__________
Is it correct to conclude that you are no longer able to have sympathy for people when you are performing your duties as a paramedic?	__________	__________
Is it correct to conclude that you are no longer able to feel any emotion for people when you are doing your paramedic duties?	__________	__________
Would you say that you are on the road to burnout?	__________	__________
Would you say that you are definitely burned out?	__________	__________

**If you answered Yes to many of these questions,
you may be a candidate for burnout.**

Is It Time For a Job Change?

Is It Time For a Job Change?

1. List the reasons why it is safe to conclude that you are not happy with your job as a paramedic.

2. It's time to find another job (career). What are your plans to make this happen?

3. How long will it take before you begin your new job?

4. What will your plans be when you do not get the new job at the time you planned to obtain it?

5. List all of the jobs that you have had prior to graduating from high school.

Is It Time For a Job Change?

6.   Which of the jobs that you had prior to graduating from high school did you enjoy more than being a paramedic?

____

____

____

____

____

7.   List all of the jobs that you had after graduating from high school up to your employment as a paramedic.

____

____

____

____

____

8.   Which of the jobs that you had after graduating from high school did you enjoy doing more than being a paramedic?

____

____

____

____

____

9.   After meditating on the jobs of your past, which one will you go back to that will take the place of your job as a paramedic?

____

____

____

____

____

10.   What will be the date that you will resign as a paramedic and begin your new job?

____

____

____

____

____

Is It Time For a Job Change?

Note: If you have decided to quit your job as a paramedic, do not continue. Make your decision known to the paramedic counselor who is conducting this course.

The Agreement

The Agreement

	Yes	No

Will you respond to all of the questions
in Session Two, Preparation for Discussion, and
Solution Finder?

Will you put some thought into your responses to the
questions in Session Two, Preparation for Discussion,
and Solution Finder?

Will you be honest in your responses to the questions
in Session Two, Preparation for Discussion,
and Solution Finder?

Will you be as detailed as possible in your responses to
the questions in Session Two, Preparation for Discussion,
and Solution Finder?

Will you write down how you truly feel in your response
to the questions in Session Two, Preparation for Discussion,
and Solution Finder?

Will you be willing to share with the Paramedic Support
Group the problems that you are having on the
ambulance?

Will you give the Paramedic Support Group the
opportunity to help you with the problems you
are having on the ambulance?

Will you participate in the Paramedic Support Group
by writing down the problems that other paramedics
are having on the ambulance?

Will you spend time thinking of personal experiences
that relate to the problems mentioned at the Paramedic
Support Group?

The Agreement

	Yes	No
Will you spend time thinking of ways to help the paramedics participating in the Paramedic Support Group with the problems they are having on the ambulance?	_______	_______
Will you write down the suggestions that the Paramedic Support Group give to you on how to handle the problems you are having on the ambulance?	_______	_______
Will you be willing to share at the First Monthly Meeting the results of using the suggestions of the Paramedic Support Group?	_______	_______
Will you at the end of this course consider becoming a paramedic counselor?	_______	_______

Note: You must answer Yes to all of these questions before going to the next session of questions. If you answer No to one or more questions, consult the paramedic counselor at this time.

Second Session of Questions

Second Session of Questions

1. List the reasons why you do not look forward to going to work to perform your duties as a paramedic.

____
____
____
____
____

2. List the reasons why you no longer enjoy helping people as a paramedic.

____
____
____
____
____

3. List reasons why you believe other paramedics do not like being your partner on the ambulance.

____
____
____
____
____

4. List the reasons why you dislike riding the ambulance.

____
____
____
____
____

5. List three recent incidents when you did not show compassion to your patients.

____
____
____
____
____

Second Session of Questions

6.   If you had to do it over again, why would you choose not to become a paramedic?

7.   Explain why you get depressed when you think about your job as a paramedic.

8.   List the reasons why being a paramedic is, to you, just a job that pays the bills and nothing more.

9.   List as many aspects of your job as a paramedic that you do not like.

10.   List the reasons why you no longer want to remain a paramedic.

Second Session of Questions

11.   Why do you get upset when citizens call for an ambulance for matters that are not an emergency?

____

____

____

____

____

12.   Why do you get impatient with patients who call on a regular basis?

____

____

____

____

____

13.   Why do you get angry with patients who wait until after 12:00 a.m. to call for matters that could have been taken care of during the daytime?

____

____

____

____

____

14.   How do you respond when the doctors and nurses are unkind or rude because you are bringing patients to their hospitals?

____

____

____

____

____

15.   Why is it difficult for you to work aggressive CPR when it is obvious (based on medical history or trauma) that life will not be restored?

____

____

____

____

Second Session of Questions

16.   Why do you complain about your job as a paramedic?

17.   List the reasons why the average person could not perform the duties of a paramedic.

18.   List the reasons why you need help with the problems you are having as a paramedic.

19.   List the aspects of the process of keeping your paramedic certification that causes you to not want to remain a paramedic anymore.

20.   There is a paramedic who does not want to ride the ambulance with you. List the reasons why you think this is so.

Second Session of Questions

21.   List the reasons why you believe a particular paramedic does not get along with you while riding the ambulance.

22.   List the reasons why you consistently don't show compassion towards your patients.

23.   List the reasons why you believe that you are burned out as a paramedic.

24.   There is a paramedic who is experiencing burnout. Why would this person not feel comfortable coming to you for help?

25.   List the things you would have to do in order to get a good night's rest prior to riding the ambulance.

Preparation for Discussion

Preparation for Discussion

1.   Write down all of the problems that you are having on the ambulance. (Be as specific as possible.)

Preparation for Discussion

2.   Write down the reasons why you no longer want to be a paramedic. Note: Once you have completed answering questions #1 and #2 let the paramedic counselor know.

Preparation for Discussion

3.   Once the paramedic counselor gives the okay, each paramedic will share with the group the problems he/she is having on the ambulance, and you will write them down.

Preparation for Discussion

4. Once the paramedic counselor gives the okay, each paramedic will share with the group the reasons why he/she no longer wants to be a paramedic, and you will write them down.

5. Based on the information shared with the Paramedic Support Group on the problems that other paramedics are having on the ambulance, you want to write down personal experiences showing that you can relate with the problems the other paramedics are having.

6. Based on the information shared with the Paramedic Support Group on the reasons for no longer wanting to be a paramedic, you want to write down personal experiences showing you can relate with others' reasons for no longer wanting to be a paramedic.

Preparation for Discussion

7. It is time for you to help the paramedics in the Paramedic Support Group with the problems they are having on the ambulance by doing the following:

    A. First, you must respond to all of the questions in the Solution Finder.

    B. After you have answered the questions in the Solution Finder, then go to #9 in Preparation for Discussion and write down potential solutions to the problems that the paramedics are having on the ambulance.

    C. Do not write down what you feel are the solutions to your personal problems on the ambulance. The other paramedics will share with you what they feel are the solutions to your problems on the ambulance. So let your focus be on helping other paramedics with their problems.

    D. Read #8 at this time.

8. It is time for you to help the paramedics in the Paramedic Support Group who no longer want to be paramedics by doing the following:

    A. First, you must respond to all of the questions in the Solution Finder.

    B. After you have answered the questions in the Solution Finder, then go to #10 in Preparation for Discussion and write down potential solutions that will help the paramedics who no longer desire to be paramedics.

    C. Do not write down what you feel are the solutions to the reasons why you no longer want to be a paramedic. The other paramedics will share with you what they feel will help you to once again desire to be a paramedic. So let your focus be on helping other paramedics.

    D. Go to Solution Finder on pages 49 – 58.

Preparation for Discussion

9. Take each problem that you heard from the other paramedics and write down solutions that you feel will help them.

Preparation for Discussion

10.   Take each reason given that you heard from the other paramedics as to why they no longer want to be paramedics and write down the solutions that you feel will help them. (Let the paramedic counselor know when you have completed this section.)

11. Once the paramedic counselor gives the okay, you will write down the solutions that each paramedic is suggesting as to how you are to handle the problems that you are having on the ambulance.

12. Once the paramedic counselor gives the okay, you will write down the solutions that each paramedic is suggesting as to how you are to handle not wanting to be a paramedic anymore.

Solution Finder

Solution Finder

Instructions:

1. These questions are to be used to help respond to sections #9 and #10 in Preparation for Discussion.

2. Keep in mind the problems other paramedics are having when responding to these questions.

3. Keep in mind the reasons the other paramedics no longer want to be paramedics while answering these questions.

4. After completing these questions, go back and respond to sections #9 and #10 in Preparation for Discussion.

Solution Finder

1.   List ways in which your duties as a paramedic can provide a sense of fulfillment.

2.   What are your commitments as a paramedic?

3.   What were your expectations of a paramedic prior to getting the job?

4.   List why you have not met the expectations of your job as a paramedic.

5.   List how you can avoid the expectations of your job as a paramedic that can lead to failure.

6.   List how you can keep from getting overly involved as a paramedic.

____
____
____
____
____

7.   Why do you believe that you should leave your work at work and not relive it again at home?

____
____
____
____
____

8.   List ways in which you can take care of yourself emotionally.

____
____
____
____
____

9.   List ways in which you can be positive about your job as a paramedic.

____
____
____
____
____

10.   How do you truly feel about your duties as a paramedic?

____
____
____
____
____

Solution Finder

11.   List the times when you can relax from your duties as a paramedic.

12.   List ways in which your peers can help with the problems you are having as a paramedic.

13.   List how you will make a difference as a paramedic.

14.   List how you would like to be shown appreciation for your job as a paramedic.

15.   List how you will show others appreciation for their jobs as paramedics.

Solution Finder

16.   List the ways in which you have handled the problems of your past.

____

____

____

____

____

17.   State how you can handle the problems of being a paramedic the same way you handled
        the problems of your past.

____

____

____

____

____

18.   List ways in which you can become a better paramedic.

____

____

____

____

____

19.   Have you admitted to the fact that you are on the road to burnout?

____

____

____

____

____

20.   Make a list of what you can eat and drink which will help you with burnout.

____

____

____

____

____

Solution Finder

55

21.   Why do you believe that your inability to share inner concerns with other paramedics led to burnout?

22.   List the names of paramedics who you can go to in order to share the problems you are having as a paramedic.

23.   List the times when you can take breaks from your duties as a paramedic.

24.   List ways in which you can take things less personally as a paramedic.

25.   What are some interests that you have outside your job as a paramedic that bring relaxation?

Solution Finder

26.   List specific goals that you have as a paramedic.

27.   List ways in which you can make your job as a paramedic more meaningful.

28.   What are some things you can do to help overcome burnout?

29.   List why you should not take on people's problems while performing your duties as a paramedic.

30.   List ways in which your duties as a paramedic can provide a sense of enjoyment.

Solution Finder

31.   List the realistic goals you have as a paramedic.

32.   List some things that you can do different that will help you with the problems of a paramedic.

33.   List ways in which you can keep from taking on the problems of your patients as your own.

34.   State how you can keep from reacting to negative comments as if they were personal insults.

35.   List ways in which you should take care of yourself physically.

Solution Finder

36.   List how you will keep your problems at work from causing problems at home.

37.   List the challenging occupations you have had in the past.

38.   State how the challenging occupations of your past can help with your experiences as a paramedic.

39.   Have you admitted that you are burned out?

40.   List the things that you can do to rest from your duties as a paramedic.

**Note: After responding to all the questions in Solution Finder,
go to sections #9 and #10 of Preparation for Discussion (pages 45-46).**

First Monthly Meeting

First Monthly Meeting

1. Share with the Paramedic Support Group the success you are having in using their suggestions on how to handle the problems you were having on the ambulance.

2. Share with the Paramedic Support Group the success you are having using their suggestions in handling your desire not to be a paramedic.

3. Write down the problems that are shared with the Paramedic Support Group that paramedics are still having on the ambulance.

4. Write down the reasons that are shared with the Paramedic Support Group concerning why they still do not want to be paramedics.

First Monthly Meeting

5.   Share with the Paramedic Support Group personal experiences that will show you can relate with the problems that the paramedics are still having on the ambulance.

6.   Share with the Paramedic Support Group personal experiences that will show you can relate with the reasons why they no longer want to be paramedics.

7.   Based on what you heard at the meeting today, share with the Paramedic Support Group your suggestions that will help them with the problems they are having on the ambulance.

8.   Based on what you heard at the meeting today, share with the Paramedic Support Group your suggestions that will help them with the reasons they no longer want to be paramedics.

9.   Write down the suggestions that the Paramedic Support Group gave to you that will help with the problems you are still having on the ambulance.

10.   Write down the suggestions that the Paramedic Support Group gave to you that will help with the reasons why you still do not want to be a paramedic.

Second Monthly Meeting

Second Monthly Meeting

1.   Share with the Paramedic Support Group the success you are having in using their suggestions on how to handle the problems you were having on the ambulance.

2.   Share with the Paramedic Support Group the success you are having in using their suggestions in handling your desire not to be a paramedic.

3.   Write down the problems that are shared with the Paramedic Support Group that paramedics are still having on the ambulance.

4.   Write down the reasons that are shared with the Paramedic Support Group of why they still do not want to be paramedics.

5.   Share with the Paramedic Support Group personal experiences that will show you can relate with the problems that the paramedics are still having on the ambulance.

Second Monthly Meeting

6.   Share with the Paramedic Support Group personal experiences that will show you can relate with the reasons why they no longer want to be paramedics.

7.   Based on what you heard at the meeting today, share with the Paramedic Support Group your suggestions that will help them with the problems they are still having on the ambulance.

8.   Based on what you heard at the meeting today, share with the Paramedic Support Group your suggestions that will help them with the reasons they no longer want to be paramedics.

9.   Write down the suggestions that the Paramedic Support Group gave to you that will help with the problems that you are still having on the ambulance.

10.   Write down the suggestions that the Paramedic Support Group gave to you that will help with the reasons why you still do not want to be a paramedic.

Third Monthly Meeting

Third Monthly Meeting

1. Share with the Paramedic Support Group the success you are having in using their suggestions on how to handle the problems you were having on the ambulance.

2. Share with the Paramedic Support Group the success you are having in using their suggestions in handling your desire not to be a paramedic.

3. Share with the Paramedic Support Group how things have improved in performing your duties as a paramedic.

4. Write down any unexpected issues / concerns that have come up that other paramedics need help with, as it relates to their job as a paramedic.

5. Share with the Paramedic Support Group your suggestions that will help the paramedics with the unexpected issues / concerns that have come up, as it relates to their job as a paramedic.

Third Monthly Meeting

6   Write down the suggestions given to you from the Paramedic Support Group that will help you with the unexpected issues / concerns that have come up, as it relates to your job as a paramedic.

7.   Share with the Paramedic Support Group specific goals you have set that will help you to be a better paramedic.

Fourth Monthly Meeting

Fourth Monthly Meeting

1.   Share with the Paramedic Support Group the progress you have made in accomplishing the specific goals you set at the Third Monthly Meeting.

2.   Share with the Paramedic Support Group the success you are having in using their suggestions on how to handle the unexpected issues / concerns that have come up, as it relates to your job as a paramedic.

3.   Share with the Paramedic Support Group why you are beginning to like your job as a paramedic.

4.   Share with the Paramedic Support Group the reasons why you are now beginning to want to remain a paramedic.

5.   Share with the Paramedic Support Group specific goals you have set that will help you to be a better paramedic.

Fifth Monthly Meeting

Fifth Monthly Meeting

1.   Share with the Paramedic Support Group the progress you have made in accomplishing the specific goals you set at the Fourth Monthly Meeting.

____

____

____

____

____

2.   Share with the Paramedic Support Group why you like your job as a paramedic.

____

____

____

____

____

3.   Share with the Paramedic Support Group the reasons why you want to remain a paramedic.

____

____

____

____

____

4.   Share with the Paramedic Support Group specific goals you have set that will help you to be a better paramedic.

____

____

____

____

____

Sixth Monthly Meeting

Sixth Monthly Meeting

1.   Share with the Paramedic Support Group the progress you have made in accomplishing the specific goals you set at the Fifth Monthly Meeting.

____

____

____

____

____

2.   Share with the Paramedic Support Group what you believe is the key to handling the problems you experienced on the ambulance.

____

____

____

____

____

3.   Share with the Paramedic Support Group why you now enjoy performing your duties as a paramedic.

____

____

____

____

____

4.   Share with the Paramedic Support Group how you are able to keep a positive attitude towards riding the ambulance.

____

____

____

____

____

5.   Share with the Paramedic Support Group the reasons why you look forward to going to work to perform your duties as a paramedic.

____

____

____

____

____

Sixth Monthly Meeting

6.   Share with the Paramedic Support Group the reasons why you are glad that you did not quit your job as a paramedic.

____
____
____
____
____

7.   Share with the Paramedic Support Group how they have been helpful to your career as a paramedic.

____
____
____
____
____

8.   Share with the Paramedic Support Group how you will use your recovery from burnout to help other paramedics.

____
____
____
____
____

The Key to the Prevention of Burnout

The Key to the Prevention of Burnout

1. **Early Action**

   A. Burnout is less likely to take place if you get a head start on it.

   B. There are many ways to cope with burnout. The same methods that are used to deal with burnout should also be used as a means of prevention. (Do not wait to become burned out before using the solutions—use them to keep from becoming burned out.)

   (Maslach, 1982, p. 132)

2. **What is the best early warning system for burnout?**

   A. You will know if you are completely burned out.

   B. However, paramedics whom you work with will probably spot the early signs of burnout in you before you do.

   C. Normally, your attention will be focused outward, toward other people and their problems, which means you will pay less attention to what you yourself are doing.

   D. You are not likely to observe the obvious change that takes place in your mood, your attitudes toward others, or your behavior on the job.

   E. If you do notice any changes, you may be inclined to deny or dismiss them as being caused by something else.

   F. This is why the best early warning system for burnout lies not in you but in other paramedics recognizing what is happening to you.

   G. In turn, you are the early warning system for other paramedics.

   (Maslach, 1982, p. 132)

3. **What does the success of an early warning system depend on in dealing with burnout?**

   The success of an early warning system depends not only on the paramedic's ability to see the warning signs in other paramedics, but also on the paramedic's willingness to speak up and say so in a supportive and constructive way.

   (Maslach, 1982, p. 132)

Are You Ready To Be a Paramedic Counselor?

Are You Ready To Be a Paramedic Counselor?

Guidelines on How To Conduct the Paramedic Support Group

1. Decide which paramedic will conduct the Paramedic Support Group.

2. The paramedic counselor must do the following **prior to conducting** the Paramedic Support Group:

   A. Read:

      1. Purpose of This Course.

      2. An Interview with the Author

      3. The Remedy to Burnout

      4. How to Use This Workbook

   B. Complete:

      1. First Session of Questions

      2. Are You a Burnout?

      3. Is It Time For a Job Change?

      4. The Agreement

      5. Second Session of Questions

   C. Read:

      Preparation for Discussion (questions #3, #4, #5, #6, #7, #8, #9, #10, #11, & #12)

   D. Complete:

      Preparation for Discussion (questions #1 & #2)

   E. Read:

      Solution Finder

Are You Ready To Be a Paramedic Counselor?

3.   Begin the course by following *The Burnout Paramedic: Remedy & Prevention* Course Outline.

Suggested Time:	Topic:
10 minutes	Purpose of This Course
	An Interview with the Author
	The Remedy to Burnout
	How to Use This workbook
20 minutes	First Session of Questions
10 minutes	Are You a Burnout?
10 minutes	Is It Time For a Job Change?
5 minutes	The Agreement
25 minutes	Second Session of Questions
30 minutes	Preparation for Discussion (questions #1, #2, #3, #4, #5, #6, #7, & #8)
30 minutes	Solution Finder
40 minutes	Preparation for Discussion (questions #9, #10, #11, & #12)
3 hours	Total Time

Are You Ready To Be a Paramedic Counselor?

4.   Specific Instructions for the Paramedic Counselor:

A.	Notes	Let the paramedics know that pages 97-112 are available if they need more room to write.
B.	Glossary	Let the paramedics know that there is a glossary on pages 87-91 for when they come to words they are not sure of the meaning.
C.	Pages 11-16	First Session of Questions

If a paramedic does not finish responding to the questions by the end of 20 minutes, tell them that they are to finish answering the questions when it is time to begin responding to the Second Session of Questions.

D.   Pages 23-26   Is It Time For a Job Change?

When paramedics inform you that they have decided to quit their jobs as paramedics:

1. Listen closely to their reasons for this decision.

2. Encourage them to continue with the course.

3. Write down on the Notes pages in the back of this book their reasons for wanting to quit so that you will be mindful of ways in which they can be helped.

E.   Pages 27-29   The Agreement

When paramedics inform you that they cannot answer Yes to all of the questions:

1. Listen closely to their reasons for this decision.

2. Encourage them to continue with the course.

3. Write down on the Notes pages in the back of this book their reasons for responding with the answer of No to the questions in this session.

Are You Ready To Be a Paramedic Counselor?

4.   Specific Instructions for the Paramedic Counselor (continued):

   F.   Pages 31-36   Second Session of Questions

           1.   Have the paramedics go back to the First Session of
                   Questions if they did not finish.

           2.   All of the paramedics must finish responding to all of the
                   questions in the Second Session of Questions before going
                   to the Preparation for Discussion.

   G.   Pages 37-48   Preparation for Discussion

           1.   Once all paramedics have completed questions #1 and #2,
                   begin questions #3 and #4.

           2.   Go to Solution Finder after completing question #8.

           3.   Once all the paramedics have completed question #10,
                   begin questions #11 & #12.

           4.   First Monthly Meeting

                   Set a date and time for the First Monthly Meeting.

5.   Monthly Meetings Course Outline

   Suggested Time: Topic:

   1 to 3 hours   First Monthly Meeting

   1 to 3 hours   Second Monthly Meeting

   1 to 3 hours   Third Monthly Meeting

   1 to 3 hours   Fourth Monthly Meeting

   1 to 3 hours   Fifth Monthly Meeting

   1 to 3 hours   Sixth Monthly Meeting

Glossary

Glossary

Abdicate	to give up; to surrender
Abstract	thought of apart from material objects; art not representing things realistically; theoretical
Accentuate	emphasize
Affection	fond or tender feeling
Alienate	to make unfriendly or withdrawn
Apathy	lack of emotion; lack of interest; listlessness
Asocial	avoiding contact with others; selfish
Bias	partiality; prejudice
Bizarre	odd
Buffer	anything that lessens shock
Buoyant	having the ability or tendency to float; cheerful
Callous	lacking sympathy and affection; unfeeling; insensitive
Catharsis	a relieving of the emotions, as through the arts or psychotherapy
Compassion	sympathy for the sorrow or suffering of others; with a desire to help
Compel	to force or get by force
Compulsive	compelling; a driving force
Concrete	specific, not general
Conflagration	large and destructive fire
Counsel	a mutual exchange of ideas, discussion, and advice
Counselor	adviser
Cruel	willing or inclined to cause suffering and pain to others; merciless; causing suffering, grief, or pain; harsh
Cynic	person who doubts the goodness of human nature and believes that all people act from selfish interests
Cynicism	the attitudes or beliefs of a cynic
De	the opposite or the reverse; an undoing, removal or removal from
Decompress	to free from pressure
Depress	to make gloomy or sad
Depression	low spirits; melancholy
Devoid	completely without; empty of

Glossary

Disenchant	to strip (someone) of pleasant illusions
Disillusion	to set free from a mistaken belief in the goodness or value of some person or thing
Dislike	to have feeling against; not like
Dismal	causing gloom or misery; dark and gloomy
Dreary	gloomy; cheerless; causing low spirits
Emotion	strong feeling; any particular feeling, such as joy, fear, etc.
Empathy	the ability to feel with another and to see the world through his eyes; identification
Enjoyment	pleasure; delight; satisfaction; pleased or gratifying possession
Enthusiasm	strong and joyous feeling of interest or admiration (for)
Evoke	to call forth; to elicit (a reaction, etc.)
Exhaustion	the draining or using up of something; condition of being worn out; extreme fatigue
Fester	to linger painfully; cause a sore feeling; rankle
Formidable	causing fear or cautious respect; hard to deal with, overcome, or accomplish
Fruition	realization or attainment; fulfillment
Frustrate	to prevent from achieving a goal or gratifying a desire; to cause to have no effect
Fulfill	to complete or accomplish; meet; satisfy; to bring about; bring to actuality; realize
Gloom	deep sadness; dejection
Glum	silent and gloomy
Gripe	to cause sharp pain in the bowels; to annoy; a complaint
Hate	to have very strong feelings against
Hostility	unfriendliness; hatred; dislike
Impatient	not patient; feeling or showing annoyance with delay, opposition, etc.
Inadvertent	due to heedlessness; unintended; thoughtless
Indifferent	neutral; unconcerned; apathetic; of no importance; average
Inherent	existing in someone or something as a natural and inseparable quality

Glossary

Intermittent	alternately starting and stopping; repeated at intervals; coming and going
Intimacy	close friendship; confidential relationship
Intimate	close; confidential; innermost; private; personal
Intractable	unmanageable; not easily controlled
Intricate	involved; complicated
Intrinsic	relating to the essential nature or makeup of a thing or person; inherent
Irresponsible	not responsible; not to be depended upon
Irritability	ease of being irritated or angered
Irritate	to make impatient or angry
Isolate	to set apart or to cause to be apart from others; to select or separate from others or from some substance
Lackadaisical	listless; lacking spark or spirit; languid
Languid	without vigor or vitality; weak; listless; indifferent
Listless	indifferent because of illness, dejection, etc.; languid
Melancholy	sad; downcast; gloomy; causing sadness or gloom; low spirits
Miserable	unhappy; wretched; causing unhappiness, trouble or annoyance
Monotonous	always the same; tiresome because of sameness
Monotony	dull sameness; lack of variety; tedious uniformity
Morose	gloomy; sullen
Objective	without bias or prejudice
Overwrought	too excited; very nervous and tense; too elaborate
Paradox	statement that seems to contradict itself but expresses an element of truth; person or thing, which seems to show contradictions
Paranoia	tendency for individuals, groups, or nations to distrust others without real cause
Pessimism	tendency to emphasize the dark and gloomy aspects of a situation, especially in a cynical way, or to predict the worst possible outcome for something
Prevent	to keep or stop from happening or doing something; hinder
Quarrel	an angry dispute, argument, or disagreement; a cause for dispute or disagreement

Glossary

Rankle	to continue to be sore and painful; to be a source of persistent mental pain and irritation
Remedy	action or method to right wrongs; to repair, make right, or correct
Resilient	recovering strength or good humor quickly; buoyant
Rude	not polite; discourteous
Self-esteem	proper respect for oneself; self-respect; too high an opinion of oneself
Sensitive	quick to be affected by external objects or conditions
Shortcomings	defect or deficiency; fault
Sullen	showing bad humor; silent because of resentfulness; sulky; gloomy; dismal
Sympathetic	understanding or sharing the same feelings
Sympathy	a sharing of another's feelings, etc.; compassion
Tedious	long and dull
Theoretical	limited to or based on theory; hypothetical
Theory	the principles of an art or science, rather than its practice
Tired	exhausted; weary; fatigued
Vicarious	endured or performed by one person in place of another; shared in by imagined participation in another's experience

References

References

Christina Maslach   *Burnout – The Cost Of Caring*

                           Prentice – Hall, Inc   1982

                           Englewood Cliffs, New Jersey 07632

                           Pg 71–85   Pg 87–128   Pg 129–141

John B. Arden Ph.D.   *Surviving Job Stress*

                           How to overcome workday pressures

                           The Career Press 2002   Franklin Lakes, NJ 07417

                           Pg 9–14   Pg 17–25   Pg 105–108

David Welch   *Beyond Burnout*

Donald C. Medeiros   *How to enjoy your job again when you've just about had enough*

George A. Tate   Prentice - Hall, Inc 1982

                           Englewood Cliff, New Jersey 07632

                           Pg 3–14

Frank Minirth M.D.   *How To Beat Burnout*

Don Hawkins, Th.M.   The Moody Bible Institute 1986

Paul Meier, M.D.   Chicago, Illinois 60610

Richard Flournoy, Ph.D.   pg 13–22   Pg 143–151

Samuel H. Klarreich   *The Stress Solution*

                           A rational approach to increasing corporate and personal effectiveness

                           Key Porter Books Limited   1988

                           Toronto, Ontario Canada M5E1R2

                           Pg 25   Pg 93–95   Pg 96–97   Pg 98
                           Pg 99–104   Pg 109–112   Pg 113–122   Pg 146–159

References

Cary Cherniss

Beyond Burnout

Helping teachers, nurses, therapists, & lawyers recover from stress and disillusionment

Routledge 1995   London EC4P 4EE

Pg 37–47   Pg 121–168

Paula Jorde

Avoiding Burnout

Strategies for managing time, space, and people in early childhood education

Acropolis Books LTD   1982

Washington, D.C. 20009

Pg 24–51

Webster's New World

Compact Desk Dictionary and Style Guide, Second Edition

Wiley Publishing, Inc. 2002   Cleveland, Ohio

The Intermediate Dictionary

Holt Rinehart Winston

NOTES

NOTES

NOTES

NOTES

NOTES

NOTES

NOTES

NOTES

NOTES

NOTES

NOTES

NOTES

NOTES

NOTES

NOTES

NOTES